Work It O

Buying a S

One woman's journey

by Jane Aireton

In a series of brief books for busy people:

Work It Out In a Week: Success At Sixty+
(with Bridget Postlethwaite)
Work It Out In a Week: Your Money
Work It Out In a Week: Christmas
Work It Out In a Week: Changing Habits

Time you old gypsy man, will you not stay,
put up your caravan just for one day?

Ralph Hodgeson

Acknowledgements

As usual, first thanks must go to my long-suffering husband Mike for putting up with my spending hours writing in the garden shed. His occasional cups of tea and glasses of wine have fuelled my creative spirit. Heartfelt thanks then go to my lovely friends both called Bridget who are my tireless editors, advisors and proof readers.

The background of the cover photo was the work of Petr Vysohlid on Unsplash cleverly adapted by Niezeka on Fiverr. Bongoneshian on Fiverr is my formatting and uploading expert who puts the show on the road.

The new component is Perran Sands Holiday Park in Cornwall. Trudy, Chris and Christine have been my mentors and have expertly guided me through the fascinating journey of buying and living in a static caravan in the beautiful dunes of North Cornwall. Thanks also go to June Donnery, General Manager of Perran Sands Holiday

Park, for supplying its fascinating inside story.

Finally, rescue dogs have played a huge part in my life. They are my faithful companions who, although they have been let down badly by the human race continue to trust and give me so much. Just as this book was going to print my little Trixie Belle slipped away leaving a huge doggy paw print on my heart. All I want to say is thank you.

Contents

Introduction

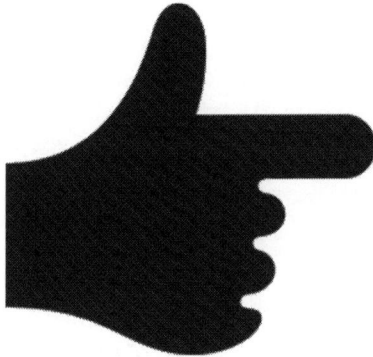

This book is not a review of static caravan parks, or indeed of static caravans, but one woman's experience of locating a park and a pitch, of finding and purchasing her van. It is about her experience of enjoying time on a park, which turned out to tick all her boxes and exceed her expectations in every direction. It is about spending time in a vibrant, positive, well-run environment that respects the earth and understands sustainability; a privilege and pleasure which are not afforded to many.

Because my home is in the Channel Islands and the park I chose was on the mainland, the Work It Out In A Week format has had to be extended - as the English Channel stands between me and my objective.

From my first thoughts, it took an hour to make the decision, thirty seconds to convince my husband, a day to research static caravans and to find the park/pitch on the Internet. On foot, it took me half a day to check out Perran Sands, a day to check out the alternatives, half an hour to review the pitch and a day to find and buy the right van plus half an hour to initiate the decking. There were several weeks separating each part of the operation and a couple of weeks before the caravan could be moved to its new site. The kitting out took a few days but I reckon this process still more than qualifies for a place on my "Work It Out In A Week" bookshelf.

Chapter 1
The Light Bulb Moment

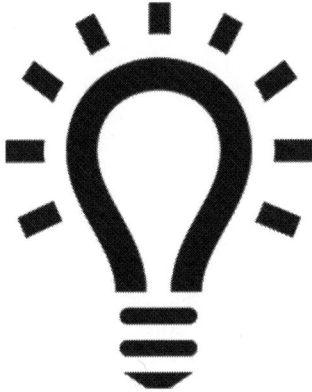

Each one of you who picks up this book will have a different reason for purchasing a static caravan. Because we are doing this journey together, I will map out for you my particular path. If you wish to go straight to the heart of the matter and are not interested in where I was coming from, jump straight to chapter 2.

Trickling rivulets chase each other down the pane as flaming June dissolves into the puddle, which is an English summer, but nothing, not even the weather, can dampen my spirits.

I have waited so long for this moment; to have an affordable place of my own by the sea where I can write, entertain my grandchildren, talk with sons and daughters-in-law and have quality time with my husband and dogs. The dream that has eluded me for many years is about to become a reality with a static caravan. Have I built that dream into an impossibly emotional edifice which, like a mirage, will dissolve in the cold light of the dawn of reality? Only time will tell. I quickly banish the thought to plunge into the unknown.

The final resolution to the conundrums which brought me to this point happened so fast it was breath-taking.

Six weeks ago, my life changed direction.

"What's the matter? "my husband's anxious face peered down at me. This is the man who if I went missing would not notice until his next meal had failed to appear; not because he doesn't care but because his mind is focussed on his next project - the latest clock he is designing or the fishing reel repair he is doing for a friend. In other words, his mind is on higher things, not what his crazy wife is doing.

Supper had not appeared and two hours later his stomach had prompted his absent mind that something must be amiss.

Not finding me in the kitchen - my natural habitat when I am not writing - he had pursued other lines of enquiry until he found me flat out in the bedroom, a place I normally only visit during the hours of darkness. Half an hour later I was in our tiny local hospital being hotwired to an ECG machine with a blood pressure of astronomic proportions.

Enter the lifestyle change.

There is nothing like a wakeup call from your heart to stimulate action. Like many women, I have been in the habit of ignoring my body's requests for rest and relaxation. As my husband says I have not been issued with an 'off switch' and constantly push myself to the limits. When my body has finally had enough and I am forced to take action, as in this case, I view chemical medicine with extreme suspicion and to be avoided wherever possible (trust me, I was a nurse). It may be a lifesaver in some cases (my husband Mike would die in three days if he didn't take his insulin) but for many it is a merely life preserver which significantly diminishes its quality. If I was to take notice of what my heart was telling me, a lifestyle change was what I needed - and fast - before I was propelled towards those magic bullets with horrible side effects.

The easy part was identifying the areas of stress that had caused these physical problems - and there were three – being a trustee of a local charitable project, the inability to sell our big house and only seeing the grandchildren for one or two weeks a year.

The next and more tricky part was how to tackle these areas. I am not a quitter and am not in the habit of letting people down but I needed to check on my priorities. If I succumbed to the stroke or heart attack to which my current medical symptoms pointed I would not only not be of use to anyone but worse still, a possible burden. Committees will carry on arguing whether you are there or not and however indispensable you may feel yourself to be, you will be amazed how well they get on without you. To your family you are different, you are their grandmother or mother, grandfather or father, brother or sister; to your friends you are special, you bring something to their lives that no one else does. You have a particular place, which needs to be protected and cherished, and is much harder to replace. If you have no family or your family doesn't appreciate you, there are plenty of people who will, so go out and find them.

My first job was to resign my trusteeship. I found it hard to let go but spending significantly large amounts of time away from home in my impending lifestyle changes would help. Did I need the status of trusteeship, did I need the work, was my contribution that important after all these years? Absolutely not and I felt immeasurably better the moment I resigned. The hole created by my resignation, like the one on the beach excavated by my dog, began to fill up with another's input. New blood began to flow in *and* I was free to move on. My blood pressure had already started to drop as relief kicked in.

The house situation was a little trickier. We had downsized to a much smaller property having taken my own advice in my first book "Work it out in a Week-Success at 60 plus" and we had hoped to sell it quickly. The solution which had suggested itself in "Work it out in a week-my money", written the previous year, had turned sour and necessitated huge amounts of work on said property. As I mentioned in that book, if the first solution doesn't work out just hunt for another, there's bound to be one just around the corner. Luckily, I had now managed to rent the house out for 6 months so for the moment the pressure off from that angle.

Finally, there was the problem of not seeing the family. This was eating me up inside. My husband and I live on Alderney, the third largest Channel Island, after

Jersey and Guernsey, and to fly to Southampton, spend all day on the train to get to the grandchildren in Cornwall is a bit of a mission and expense besides which there are the dogs to consider. Our dogs are both rescue animals and hate going into kennels as they feel they are back in the pound. This means dogs sitters living in, with more upset for them and more expense for us.

For many years I had been looking after older family members and was stuck like a limpet to the rock. Now I was free but tied by property and the resultant lack of funds. The time had come to break loose.

To retain our Channel Island residential status, and as Mike wants to live on Alderney forever, meant that we could only stay away from the island for 90 days. We could not afford yet another property and the sale of the big house was to provide our income. My plan had been to build a tiny house, a romantic notion, but not, as my husband tactfully pointed out, a very practical one.

I had drooled over pictures of cabins in the woods far away from the hustle and bustle, imagined leading the simple life playing with my grandchildren and getting back to basics. Where would I site it? Far away from the hustle and bustle meant that anyone with enough ingenuity could tow it away undisturbed by neighbours. Even if my sons had a suitable garden or fields, (which they didn't), being right on top of them was not a plan.

Worse than that I had built up my tiny house expectations to fever pitch and had gone so far as to check out suppliers. However, on arriving at the premises of the company I had thought might supply the parts for said van, I was met by a man who had either lost a close relative very recently or lacked an ability to respond to other forms of human life. It was a bitingly cold day in February and together with his two workmates he stared morosely at me answering my excited questions with monosyllables. The tiny home he had on view was depressing in the extreme with the bathroom cladding peeling off, as he had prepared it in a hurry for an exhibition. A candelabra swung disconsolately above the bed space and my excitement evaporated in an instant. My break for freedom now seemed further away than ever, on all counts.

Fast forward to my cardiac incident.

Lying in bed rearranging my life in my head, I idly typed the word 'caravan' into the Google space bar. Up came 'caravan parks'. Suddenly sparks seem to go off in my limpid brain and I sat up and began typing words in furiously. Why had I not thought of that before? Only once had I stayed in a tiny caravan park and it had been a very pleasant experience. OK, the word 'static' as applied to caravans in such parks does not fit either my personality or activities, but it was only a word after all's said and done and if that word was going to get me where I wanted to be, I could live with that.

Static caravans might look identical on the outside, but inside I could create magic to my heart's content. Suddenly a new line of enquiry opened before my very eyes. My tiny house idea was a beautiful dream but in my case, it just wasn't going to happen.

The buffers of life were beginning to loom large and dreaming wasn't going to get me where I needed to be. A little metal box by the sea suddenly seemed incredibly attractive. Maybe it was an affordable way to get to where I wanted to go? Maybe, just for once, the light at the end of my tunnel was not an oncoming train?

Chapter 2
The Research

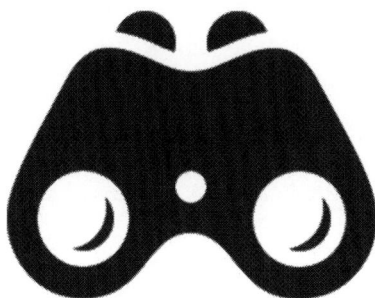

Having latched onto THE IDEA, it was time to collect data. Resting in bed was an ideal time to drift around the Internet, not so much surfing as belly-boarding. 'Static' was not a word that described anything I had ever done but if I was going to make this happen I had to accept that it was the name of the game. Going to a park meant that I had a pitch that was monitored all year round and the wagon of my dreams could not be removed in the dead of night.

I was of, course, looking for a holiday park and as such it would probably be closed during the winter and not suitable as a permanent residential address, but that suited me fine.

Obviously the first consideration was where I wanted to be. It was easy for me to select a park as the criteria were clear cut; it needed to be about half an hour from my boys and their families on the North Cornish coast. For most people, the choice of park tends to be within easy reach of home so they can visit it on a regular basis.

The next consideration was what the park needed to contain. Would you be looking for peace and quiet with fishing lakes? Would you be looking for amusements for a young family? What are your criteria? In my case I needed a dog-friendly park with peace and quiet, plus entertainments for the young, no fishing lakes required.

Another important consideration is the surrounding area and in my case, I wanted a beach and plenty of countryside to explore. With family close by, I was not too dependent on interesting places to visit, although the mouth-watering PYO Trevaskis fruit farm proved very attractive and the fact that the Eden project, the Lost Gardens of Heligan, and the Minack theatre were all in the vicinity were by no means inconsequential. They were added bonuses rather than the raison d' être.

Whilst looking for holiday parks in North Cornwall, of which there are many in the Newquay area, almost immediately Perran Sands Park run by Haven caught my eye. It appeared to provide the combination of peace and quiet and activity for the grandchildren for which I was searching. There was the beach I wanted (although it turned out to be quite a trek to get to it) and an indoor and outdoor swimming pool on site. In any event there was an easily accessible beach at Perranporth three minutes away.

The number of poo bins, indicated on the map of the park, made it quite clear that it was a dog-friendly site with lots of easy dog (and child) walks close by in the dunes. There was a restaurant, a fish and chip shop and a Pizza parlour onsite, plus a variety of activities aimed at the young.

Perran Sands quite simply ticked all the boxes.

Obviously, I needed to look at others but Perran Sands had already stolen my heart. Late that night I sent, via www.myholidaycaravan.co.uk_ (which is a brilliant site for all things static) enquiries to various sites in the area and I held my breath.

Next morning, first thing, the phone rang,

 "Trudy here…." Trudy, Trudy who? I didn't know any Trudys, I had never even met a Trudy,
"…..you enquired about Perran Sands."

Light dawned,

"Gosh that was quick. I think I want to buy a van on your park. I know nothing about static caravans and parks so you will have to guide me through."

By the end of the conversation I felt I had known Trudy all my life. Despite the fact I could only afford a very modest van, she gave me the Rolls-Royce treatment and guided me through the intricacies of owning a caravan. I could buy a new or a second-hand one on the park from Haven, or I could purchase one from an owner selling privately on the park. I would buy the van and rent the pitch.

By the end of the conversation I was all ready to jump on a plane and complete the operation but there were things to be done. I needed to access funds and persuade my husband that this was a good idea and, in any event, Trudy was going on holiday. I had a small inheritance put aside for a rainy day, could I get hold of it now? As far as I could see the rain was lashing down in torrents and the rainy day had arrived in the form of my cardiac problems.

Trudy went on to tell me that a lady who had previously had a caravan on the park for 20 years still visited them and brought them cakes, so people obviously bonded with the park if that is what they wanted to do. She also said that owners were welcome to have a coffee and use the wi-fi in the Owners official office at any time and that the staff were always on hand to sort out problems as they arose. It appeared both well organised and friendly at the same time. We made an appointment for two and a half weeks' time and, in the meantime, I was to email her with any queries that came to mind. I discovered later that she answered those queries sitting on a deck chair in Cyprus on her holiday, such was her commitment to the job.

"Calm down Jane," I told myself as I got off the phone, "nothing is ever quite that good. In twenty-four hours, you have decided to change your lifestyle and found the park of your dreams." I had studied the park map on the website until I knew it by heart and had already found the pitch that I wanted in a tiny cul-de-sac in the dunes with a caravan on it at the right price. Would it still be available when I made it down to Cornwall for the big decision?

Belly-boarding across the Internet, I found two people selling their caravans privately on the Perran Sands site and decided to contact them to find out precisely what their costs were and what living on the park was like. This was a useful exercise and gave me lots of valuable information. It is one thing to have an average figure and quite another to have the actual costs for a given make of van. One contact was so enthusiastic that he even sent me photos of sunsets over Perran Sands and his family in the van. These owners explained that on some sites there is a certain time after which you must move your caravan on. On Perran Sands, unless the caravan was in poor condition, it could stay there for as long as you wanted. The reasons these individuals were selling were not to do with the quality of the pitch or the park but were domestic ones. Sites do not always allow you to sell privately and, although at this stage the last thing I was thinking about was selling, one always needs to know the parameters of an exit strategy.

The other sites I contacted, took longer to respond but I fixed appointments with them, as a comparison. I have to say that this was a very half-hearted attempt at making a choice.

Voraciously I devoured all the information I could about owning a caravan; the Kindle edition of "*Buying a Static Caravan*" by J. Towner was excellent and http://www.myholidaycaravan.co.uk/ filled in all the gaps. I went through a detailed comparison of caravan manufacturers, comparing size, layout, price, interior décor, build quality, etc. and, having read until my head was reeling with facts, the bottom line was that overall the major caravan manufacturers are all very similar.

The size and accommodation was critical, for me. In my price range, they all seemed in the region of 35' x 12'. I needed three bedrooms, a double for us, a girls' twin and a boys' twin for the grandchildren and two loos, including one with a shower. Luckily Mike and I get on well in confined spaces but I do not like rolling over my spouse to get out of bed so there needed to be adequate access to the double bed from both sides. As our two rescue dogs would be coming with us, Trover, a staffie with a harelip and Trixie Belle, a very old Bedlington cross poodle with attitude, there needed to be plenty of space. Double glazing was essential as, although Perran Sands is closed from the first of November to the end of February, there can be chilly days at any time of year. Central heating was also said to be essential but I was told later that a good gas fire in the lounge and heaters in the bedrooms and shower room are quite adequate. This system is also apparently less expensive to run, especially since the park is closed in the coldest months of the year. I have yet to test this statement. The van I ultimately chose does not have central heating.

My running costs would comprise:
Pitch rent (which would be reduced if I had bought a van from the park)
Electricity
Gas
Insurance
Rates (non-domestic and water/sewerage charges)
Safety inspections of gas and electricity
Alarm costs
An optional drain down charge to prevent burst pipes in freezing weather

It is advisable to make sure the park you choose is a member of the National Caravan Council, which has protocols of best practice to protect both the owner and the park operator.

A few days before I flew, the caravan and pitch of my dreams disappeared from the Perran Sands website. I was devastated. I knew it was all too good to be true.

Chapter 3
The Choice

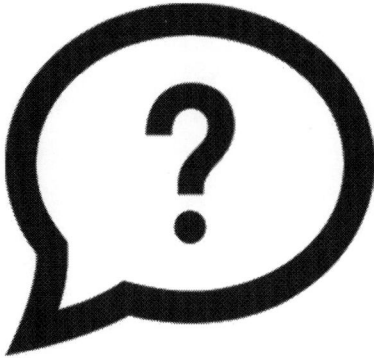

As I flew over the Needles on the Isle of Wight, en route to Southampton Airport, one sunny Friday morning, the enormity of what I was doing suddenly hit me. A caravan is not a financial investment, it depreciates year on year. We hadn't sold our big house and the money I was spending on this van was our security blanket; I was spending my inheritance to be with my grandchildren. Mike was trusting me to make good decisions whilst he looked after the dogs back on Alderney.

Trundling along in the train through Dorset, Somerset, Devon and finally Cornwall I wondered about the second-hand red Citroen 2 my younger son had picked up for me - little did I know it would shed its silencer even before I had a chance to drive it!

Luckily, my daughter-in-law, Rhalina, had agreed to come and look at the sites, pitches and vans with me to make sure I didn't get carried away. A second pair of eyes and ears is always useful when making big decisions in unknown territory. Perran Sands had offered me a very generous voucher towards lunch on Sunday so I could arrange for the whole family to view the park. Although they were all living locally, they had never visited the facility.

I arrived late on Saturday night at my younger son's house, desperate to have a quick look at the park. I had already arranged another restaurant for the following day if Perran Sands wasn't up to scratch. After a short discussion, it was decided that we had time to take a brief view of the park and I could hardly contain my excitement as we swept out of Perranporth and up the hill to our destination. To my relief if was just as I had hoped, wide open spaces and sand dunes everywhere. We parked up easily and made for the Surf Bay restaurant. It was spacious and airy with a VW camper van called Alfie right in the middle in which you could have meals if you so desired. It was perfect. As the sun began to set we sipped our drinks and wondered about the future. So far, so good.

On Sunday morning, I popped into the 'Owners' exclusive office' to pick up my meal voucher. I explained about my disappointment at missing the pitch on Piran Point to the lovely sales manager Christine, as Trudy was still in Cyprus. I learned that the park was so popular that by mid-June there would be a waiting list for pitches and the area I had chosen was particularly popular.

"You are not going to believe this," said Christine handing me the voucher, "a pitch came up yesterday in that area, so if you want to go and look at it and like it, you can put a deposit on it. I have other people coming in later today, so don't hang about. I know you are looking at other parks so if you decide against Perran Sands or you want another pitch, that deposit is fully refundable. I know you are looking at vans here on Tuesday and other places tomorrow so we will hold it until then, if you want it."

I could not believe my ears, things were falling into place yet again. The sign in my kitchen reads 'Only dead fish go with the flow' and for so many years I seem to have been struggling upstream. Maybe I was turning into a dead fish at long last and I had never wanted to be a dead fish more than at that moment.

Lunch was a blur and as soon as I could extricate myself from the family, Tom, my younger son and I hit the trail for the pitch. After five minutes' brisk walk we rounded a corner and arrived at Piran Point and our little cul-de-sac (yes, I had already mentally taken possession) nestled in the dunes. The perfect place for a pitch I would say. I was backed up against a dune, and yes, there were other vans on both sides and opposite, screened by grassy bushes, but here, I was tucked away from the action and protected from the storms.

One thing I checked immediately was my mobile phone signal in case of medical emergencies. I could easily get a signal, fifty yards down the road - and in fact once I got the van you could get a signal by standing on the steps just outside the front door. There was no wi-fi on the park as a whole but I could get it from the Owners' office and, quite frankly, I didn't want to be at everyone's beck and call once I was in Cornwall. I discovered later that some people use dongles but I am not sure they would work in our grassy hollow. The fact that no post could be delivered to the van was another plus for me, I wanted as little contact with the outside world as possible. Trudy later allowed me to have an outside bench delivered to the van as a one-off special concession as we lived overseas.

Climbing up the dunes opposite, Tom and I gazed across miles of dune land and identified St Piran's enormous cross. St Piran is the patron saint of tin miners, or tinners as they are known. He was apparently evicted from Ireland with a millstone around his neck and washed up at Perranporth. Noticing that his black hearthstone (ore) oozed a silver substance (tin) when heated he is credited with discovering tin smelting.

Away in the distance I could almost make out St Piran's oratory which has been covered and uncovered with sand many times over the centuries. There would certainly be plenty to explore. Around our feet twirled little blue butterflies, black and red moths, bumble bees and a myriad of insects which in our eagerness to see the bigger picture had been overlooked.

Soon it was time for the other family members to pass an opinion on the pitch, but *I* knew I had found my final resting place. I rushed back to the office, put down the deposit and returned to one of the playparks where the children were playing to their hearts' content. We all discussed the pros and cons of Granny Jane and Grandad Mike setting up in a static caravan in Perran Sands, at Piran Point, or as we now call, it Sandy Hollow. There didn't seem to be any cons so the motion was carried unanimously.

By now it seemed unnecessary to visit the other parks the next day, but it had to be done to make it feel like an informed decision. It gave us a yardstick with which to compare Perran Sands but once the day was over, Rhalina and I agreed that what had been a definite choice in my mind had now become set in stone. All that was left to do was to find the ideal caravan.

By now we had looked at a few show caravans at both at Perran Sands and the other parks which had given me a chance for comparisons. I discovered that I wasn't interested in the more elaborate and expensive ones; what I was buying was a lovely tin box, not an apology for a bungalow. I already had a proper bungalow back home.

I could scarcely sleep that night; the final piece of the jigsaw was just waiting to be placed in the puzzle.

Perran Sands already felt like home when we arrived at the 'Owners' exclusive office' next morning ready for the final choice of van, and here at long last was Trudy. She was just as I had imagined she would be. Larger than life, she oozed infectious enthusiasm for her job from every pore. Nothing was too much trouble for her and problems simply dared not venture into her territory.

I was so glad that my daughter-in-law was with me as information flowed like a waterfall, both from Trudy and Chris Chicken who handles owner admin and sales reception. They took us through every detail you could imagine and more. I was desperate to see the vans in my price range but quite rightly I had to have all the information first.

Being the sort of person who tries out a new gadget and then reads the instructions, I wasn't feeling very patient. My mind wandered out of the window and down to our perfect pitch and out into the dunes until suddenly the flow of information stopped as quickly as it had started and we were on our feet again and heading out of the office.

Because I was at the bottom end of the price range and the criterion was simple (three bedrooms, a loo and a loo plus shower) the choice was basically one second-hand van and one new one. We first looked at several new vans to ensure that I really didn't need opening French windows at one end as well as a side door, and chairs rather than stools in the eating area. Given my pitch position, which was backed up hard against the dunes and opened onto the road at the front, I didn't have a magnificent view through French windows to gaze upon and stools would do us fine. If I was going to sit outside the van it would be at the side on a bench and because there were windows on both sides of the van there would be lots of air flowing through even on the hottest day and being right by the sea there would almost always be a breeze.

The choice between buying a new or old van is a difficult one. On Perran Sands, if you buy new you can rent it out through Haven for the first seven years to offset the cost of the pitch. If you buy a second-hand or 'pre-loved' van, a somewhat pretentious expression in my view, you can rent it out for fewer years. If you buy new the depreciation is eye-watering, less so for a second-hand van but buying a caravan is not an investment in financial terms, it depreciates come what may. For me the investment was the ability to see my family and to recharge my batteries and that was an investment worth making.

The other major factor was that I didn't know how it would work out and my budget was tight. I was not looking to upgrade in the near future, which might have been easier financially had I bought a new van. Very importantly, I could get more space for my money with a second-hand van. After three years (it was a four-year-old van we were going to look at) I could still rent it out privately if that was what I wanted to do, provided it was still in good condition.

With all these facts swimming round in my head I tried to remember the perceived wisdom that the pitch (can be changed) and the park (difficult to change unless I went to another Haven park) are more important than the van. I needed to remember that I had already sorted those things in a couple of days so the purchase of my little tin box, however complicated it might seem at this moment, was the final and least important hurdle.

I could have visited the annual static caravan exhibition at the NEC and made more enquiries; I could have done much more research; but to find a park in the right place with people I trusted to point me in the right direction was good enough for me.

A holiday park is a business and to be successful it must run at a profit, so any decisions will be weighted in favour of the park. If I had bought a van on e-Bay and put it in my back garden, things would have been a fraction of the cost. What I was buying into here was a complete setup with all facilities; gardening, sub-letting, security, entertainment, the list was endless.

The second-hand van proved to be a four-year-old Willoughby Salsa Eco. Outside the van seemed in good condition, no ripples or gaps anywhere in the skin.

The big plus in buying from the site was that I knew the van's history - one careful owner - and I could be pretty sure it hadn't been damaged from being moved from pillar to post. Confidently, I had expected that as I set foot through the door I would feel an immediate affinity. Neither Rhalina nor I felt anything at all.

As Trudy took us over the features, I could do no more than miserably survey the scene. Something was not right and I couldn't place it. The accommodation was exactly what I wanted, the condition was immaculate, it was everything I had hoped for it, it just felt wrong. I could see my daughter-in-law was feeling the same.

There were no smells or signs of damp or water ingress and the upholstery was in immaculate condition; no sign of mould anywhere. The humidity had clearly been kept under control and the van well cared for. There was even an extra coat cupboard for wellies, shoes, mops and brushes just inside the door, which would be brilliantly handy.

We decided to think about what we had seen over lunch and return, hopefully with a clearer head, after we had eaten. Were we exhausted by information overload and the impending decision? There seemed no logical reason why it didn't seem right.

We sat in the lovely Surfbay Restaurant and considered what had happened. Neither of us could work out what was going on, why didn't it seem right. We went back and revisited the new van we had been shown in the Show Park, but that quite definitely wasn't right. The only course of action open to us was to have another viewing of the second-hand Salsa later in the afternoon.

Trudy patiently drove is back to the pre-loved van whose owners were upgrading. We all agreed it fitted the bill, especially seeing that it had a pitched roof to accommodate tall people, both my sons being well over six feet tall. It also had an extra double bed, which you could unroll from the seating in the cabin, for extra-long guests or someone in a wheelchair. We couldn't find one reason why it wouldn't be ideal. All in all, although it was not love at first sight, we decided it was the way to go and so the deal was sealed there and then.

Chris and Trudy now presented me with a comprehensive folder of information to digest. Here are some examples of the contents.

1. A holiday home service and repair charter, with guaranteed time scales for diagnosing and fixing problems, which was essential if I was to be renting the caravan out.

2. Details about how to over-winter my van to prevent burst pipes.

3. Insurance details. I could probably have found a cheaper insurance elsewhere but doing it through Haven made sense as we were so far away and any claims could be dealt with quickly on the spot.

4. Details of the Ramtech security system installed in the van, which alerts a member of the security team 24/7 if activated. This was important to me being in a remote part

of the park and only expecting to be on site three months of the year.

5. The NCC code of practice. The NCC is the UK trade body for the holiday park industry. The code of practice is primarily for the benefit and protection of holiday homeowners and sets out principles of good practice.

It would be a couple of weeks before the van could be moved to its new pitch, as it had rental guests booked in for the next week. I agreed to return with my husband to take control of the keys once it was in position and we would spend a week 'on board,' nest-building and getting to know the territory.

Many finance deals are available when buying a van but I had been left that small inheritance and wanted to tie the deal up there and then. Overall, I never felt any sales pressure. Trudy had immediately grasped what I wanted and didn't waste time showing us vans that were not suitable to my needs or putting pressure on me to buy a new van.

To buy second-hand through the park seemed sensible as I was the new girl on the block and if I bought privately then I had to rely on the honesty of the owner. Also, one of the caravans I had considered privately was let for most of the summer already, and I wanted the van immediately, if not sooner.

That night, sitting down with a glass of wine and surrounded by my family, I wondered what on earth I had just done and what the future would hold. Would Mike approve of my purchase, how would we deal with the dogs? I hadn't checked for rust on the chassis or whether the pipes were lagged and once moved I must check that it had four chains holding it down - but that was all for another day. No longer a limpet on the Alderney rock, I now had one foot very firmly in a little tin box in a sand dune in north Cornwall.

Chapter 4
The Reality
(or 7 days on site)

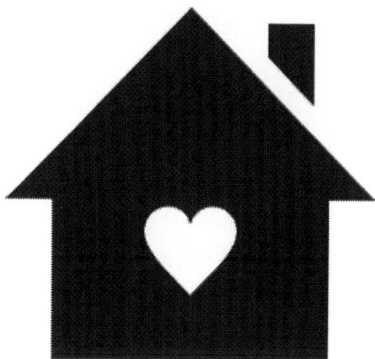

I must remember never put my lovely gentle husband Mike and Dr Death, the voice on my GPS, together in a car. It will always end in tears.

To say that my sense of direction is poor is the understatement of the year and so, approaching Perran Sands to show Mike how I have spent our financial buffer, I elect to use Dr Death to help me get there. It doesn't help that I have started out from my elder son's house on the top of a hill miles from anywhere and for some reason Dr Death can't locate his satellites.

In desperation Mike pulls out the map and the contest begins. What I had envisaged as mounting excitement and enthusiasm for my new venture was more like,
" Well, I have no idea where we are."
"I am sure I went this way last time and the satellites were available then."
"Well why do you need me and Dr Death, neither of whom have the faintest idea where we are?"
"I just didn't want to make any mistakes," I end, feebly wishing I could have remembered the route more clearly.
Suddenly, without warning, Dr Death finds his satellites and we are back on track, but the damage is done. Mike angrily stuffs the map in the glove box and we approach our destination with a distinct air of tension in the car.

As we turn the corner into the long winding drive of Perran Sands, I switch off Dr Death and can feel my shoulders begin to relax; I know I am home. Six weeks ago, I didn't know this place existed, now it has become a place where I can shed all my burdens, spend time with my family, write in peace and nest-build to my heart's content. I cautiously glance at Mike, but he never gives anything away, so I will have to wait and see what his reaction is going to be.

Although it is late on a Saturday afternoon, Trudy is waiting to greet us. It had been a long day; a flight to Southampton, four trains and two car rides but at last we are here. We have a welcome cup of tea and Mike is introduced to the staff. The first thing to be done is to have photos taken for our 'Owners Privilege Card', which will entitle us to free swimming, half price activities and 15% off in the shops and restaurants on site, plus some privileges on other sites.

We fill in eight more cards for family and friends. There are also selected establishments in Perranporth that will give us 15% off any goods or services we purchase from them. Our photographs reveal two rather bedraggled wrecks, but as long as the cards work, that is all I care about and away we drive in convoy with Trudy to our perfect pitch.

Parking up Nellie, our little red Citroen 2, in the space between our van and the next, we follow Trudy as she opens up and explains all the final details of our new home - stop cocks and security systems, heaters and vents. This is Mike's territory, I can now relax and unwind. I am relieved to see that he approves straight away. It was three days later that he discovered the third bedroom!

I had brought provisions for the journey as, with Mike being an insulin-dependent diabetic, I always need to have food available. The squashed remains of lunch do not look appealing, so we wend our weary way over to the restaurant and tuck into a delicious meal. Picking up a bottle of wine from the mini market on the way home we stroll back to the van admiring the sun setting over the dunes and fall into bed dreaming of the fun-filled days to come.

Not having a swimming pool at home on Alderney, my first priority after a good night's sleep in our very comfortable double bed, is to head off to the pool. 8.00 - 9.30 is the time allocated to owners only and I am determined to take this opportunity. Having made Mike a cup of tea in bed I take the brisk five-minute walk to the pool, where it is obviously the time for lane swimming, which suits me down to the ground.

The pool building is light and airy and, as I splash up and down in the slow lane, the intense brigade fly past creating an impression. There are two other pools for small fry and, later in the week, I would watch the lifeguards skilfully manoeuvring someone into the accessible access chair for those less physically able.

The park seems very well set up for wheelchair users with plenty of turning space both in the restaurant and pool and I later learn that specially adapted caravans are available to rent for those who need more space.

The outdoor pool is closed as the air temperature is still low at 8.30am in early June and the pool water temperature still

43

lower I would guess. Palm trees grow out of the centre of this attractive kidney shaped amenity, which has a ramped access at the shallow end. There is also an Owner's gym, which I have yet to sample!

Having swum to my heart's content I return to housekeeping duties. The van was sold to us equipped with almost everything you could possibly need, from an electric kettle and microwave to a tin opener and potato masher, but I know there will be a small list of 'extras' we will decide to buy.

The oven seems brand new, as is the fridge and the TV. I have never had a cooker hood and, having always wanted one, I am delighted to find I have one, probably very important in such a confined space. I have brought some linen and towels with me, only in modest quantities as I knew we would have to heave all our baggage on and off public transport en route and there was a 15-kg luggage allowance on the flight. I decide that all future guests should bring their own duvet cover or sleeping bag, pillow case and towels but I will provide a sheet for each bed; an item for the shopping list.

It becomes obvious I will need a front door mat and loo brushes, kitchen towel holder, dishcloths, tea towels and a potato peeler of the design I prefer. I had brought microfibre hand towels from home, one of which could double as a bath mat. I know that the worst thing in a caravan is condensation so everything I use needs to be quick drying.

The caravan comes complete with an adequate airing rack, which hangs out of the window and for which I had bought pegs. I knew that a washing line was verboten. The launderette facilities on site would prove to be good - except that later in the week I managed to put my token in one drier and my clothes in another! Luckily that was easily rectified. Tokens are available in the mini market with a 50% discount for caravan owners and I like the fact that the launderette is open from first thing until ten o'clock at night, as washing is not something I want to be doing in the middle of the day. I had thought about purchasing a caravan table-top washer/spin drier but for now I decide to stick to the launderette.

Net curtains have never been my preference but it had become obvious in the first twenty-four hours that, with the close proximity of the neighbouring vans, I would need something for privacy. Onto the shopping list go the dreaded nets. A trip to Falmouth is now clearly called for. This was before I discovered the wonderful hardware shop close by in Perranporth, but I don't think even they would have been able to provide nets.

A handy town close to the park of your choice is very useful and Perranporth being three minutes door to door provided everything from a small tool kit and drill to dressmakers' pins and lengths of chain to secure the benches. Ah yes, the outdoor benches. These are the handy plastic ones with integral storage. I had ordered one straight away as I knew I always need extra storage, even though the seats in the cabin are hollow. I knew these benches were allowable on site as many caravans had them and Trudy provided me with the relevant website from which to make the purchase.

Unknowingly, my younger son had also bought me one, as a housewarming present, so I am in seventh heaven with two. A tool kit now becomes essential for my poor husband, as he now has two benches to assemble and attach to the caravan and this is just for starters. Mike wanted to call our house at home 'Kudujus' or "Could you just..." as he is incredibly handy and is always being asked to fix things, particularly by me. It is proving to be business as usual, even down in Cornwall.

The groundsmen endlessly strim the park, especially between the caravans so Trudy had pointed out that the benches would need to be raised above ground level. As the plastic aged, it might be damaged by gardening activities - such is the attention to detail at Perran Sands.

The afternoon in Falmouth is great and at Trago Mills we pick up all we need at very reasonable prices, including the dreaded nets. After a long discussion in the fabric department I decide on butterfly decorated nets and to make the ghastly things look as good as I can, I decide on a very labour-intensive way of putting them up, in view of the fact that I don't have a sewing machine. I decide to pleat them and attach them to the van with Velcro just below the curtain rail. This would replace the conventional wire arrangements, which do not give a very pleasing result, to my way of thinking. I will stick hooked Velcro on the wall and sew fuzzy Velcro to the curtains.

I leave Mike in the second-hand bookshop whilst I trawl the charity shops for bargains; it is such fun looking at the choice, which just isn't available on our small island. I later discover that the best charity shop of all is in Perranporth. Having driven through that town on several occasions in the past, it had never appealed to me in the way, for example, that St Agnes is pretty. However, now it comes to finding what we need for the van, it has a surprisingly comprehensive mix of resources from veterinary services to and excellent delicatessen.

There was even a seamstress at Quackers Sewing Service who could make up curtains in the new colour scheme for me if I ran out of steam and who generously donated me the few extra conventional hooks I needed for the curtains. Some of the curtains were on strange devices I had not seen before that slid over the top of the rails, but Perranporth Hardware came up with the goods yet again, when I needed just a few more to make the curtains hang perfectly.

I am going to work hard on personalizing our van, as all the vans are much the same on the outside and the inside for that matter. I shall be bringing the dogs over next time so I am going to be making covers for all the seating as I am afraid our dogs think they have as much right to chairs as humans. I fancy a bit of bunting here and there and, judging by a quick peek at You Tube, it looks as though it is not too difficult to make up. Whilst in Falmouth I pick up plenty of tape on which to sew the triangles of blue fabric, as blue and white is going to be my colour scheme for the interior.

Many years ago, I helped Mike's cousin develop the Trover drying coat for dogs, which will now be invaluable in the confined space of the van. It wicks the water away from the dog's coat and is a boon when they have been in the sea or when the heavens open unexpectedly, http://www.trovercoats.com.

Most dogs don't need coats but they DO need to dry off quickly particularly in a caravan. Because the coat fixes around the dog's back legs rather than under the belly, the Trovercoat stays in position and isn't uncomfortable for the dog to stay in for extended periods. Now you know why my staffie is called Trover; he is the company mascot!

Somehow, I seem to have strayed from the subject of Day 1 in 'the van' so now to return to the matter in hand. I hope by the time I get to the end of this book I shall have developed a name for our little tin box. Nellie was an easy name for the car as the registration was NLY. As van names, I quite liked 'Adventure before Dementia' and 'The Bolt Hole' as it reflects Mike's engineering skills but nothing has struck a definitive chord yet. My quest for the definitive name continues.

Back at the van things are beginning to look a lot like home. Cases have been unpacked and stowed under the bed. The van has been equipped with some coat hangers, and I had brought some more to swell the ranks, so the ample wardrobe space is now almost full. I decide that the grandchildren can create pictures to decorate the walls so I will be keeping a lookout for frames in charity shops. All the family are very artistic - except for me - so that will be just fine.

As the sun goes down behind the dunes on Day 1 I have honestly never felt so happy. The older grandchildren are coming for a sleepover at the weekend and all is set for an amazing week.

Day 2

Day 2 is spent getting to grips with the dreaded nets. The pleating plan is beginning to look good. My ideas are generally sound but, unfortunately, I don't always envisage the amount of work involved to bring them to fruition. By the end of the holiday I will have a permanent hole in the end of one of my fingers - a repetitive needle injury. I have five small windows and one triple size window to curtain and it is certainly a case of blood, sweat and tears. The blood must be kept from the white nets at all costs. With this system, I figure that we come to leave it will be easy to take down the curtains leaving a tidy strip of white Velcro on the van.

I want to talk to Trudy about letting out the van between this visit and the next in mid-August. She explains that any rental money accrued will reduce next year's pitch rent. The park is so popular that within twenty-four hours of my request being made, seeing that it was high season, practically every week is booked, halving next year's pitch rental.

The park makes sure that the van is kept in good condition, handles the rentals and replaces any breakages of standard equipment. You are advised to take out an insurance for mattresses etc damaged during a rental period. The park will guarantee to take the high season weeks whether they are booked or not.

You are not encouraged to leave anything of value for the holiday tenants who will provide all their own laundry, towels etc. Before you return, Haven will do a free carpet and upholstery clean. Your letting calendar is available on the owner's website so if you suddenly want to use the van on a free week or book in a friend you can do just that.

I am very keen to acquire an outside deck for many reasons, not least of which it would make an exterior space for the dogs, provide an extra outdoor room and most importantly provide ramped access for many of my friends and family who are elderly or have accessibility issues.

In my part of the park, Piran Point, decks, Trudy had explained, were only available on production of a blue disabled badge. I had brought with me the relevant paperwork and headed for the "Owners exclusive office" to discuss the subject. As usual, in a flash the whole thing is arranged.

Basically, the deck will be made by a local contractor in natural wood; comprising a ramp with a gate at the top, by the door to the caravan, and a square area on which to sit and in my case to house my two benches. The hidden advantage is a storage area beneath the sitting area which will accommodate much of the gear that I do not wish to drag back to the islands with me.

Within twenty-four hours it has been priced, an equivalent pointed out to me on the self-same van as mine, the OK had been given and it has been ordered. It will be constructed, delivered and installed before I return in a couple of months' time. Trudy promises to send me a photo as soon as it had been completed. The speed, efficiency and ease with which things happen at Perran Sands is barely believable.

Day 3

The weather remains warm and calm, which makes settling in that much easier. By now several of the nets are up and I am feeling a bit less like a goldfish in a bowl.

The benches are assembled, attached to the van with little chains, and beginning to fill with belly boards and balls, charcoal and a BBQ.

I had found a camping shop in Falmouth with a sale on, which was to me simply irresistible. I picked up a little portable BBQ, heavily reduced, which we could use either outside the caravan or to take up into the dunes for a BBQ picnic. It was cunningly packaged in a canvas bag which made it eminently portable with a separate zipped section in the middle in which you could carry your meats; I love eating outdoor or 'en plein air', as the French romantically express it.

I also picked up two collapsible water bottles with carabiners on them, which proved very valuable. When full you can stand them up and then clip them to the outside of your rucksack so they don't leak on the lunch or take up valuable space. When empty you can roll them up and stow them away. Filling them from the tap means not using the dreaded plastic bottles that are polluting our oceans.

By now it is obvious that the decking is going to have a further function. The grass around the caravan has been strimmed and with the dew night and morning, it is getting walked straight into the van. Having a ramp will help to disperse the grass before any feet get as far as the door. It will also make it easier to take off shoes before entering. Under the present arrangements shoes tend to fall through the steps as one balances precariously on one leg - unless your yoga certificate is up to date - in which case you can stand there all day.

The Haven parks are incredibly well kept as I have already mentioned. At Perran Sands the ten-strong maintenance and ground work team start work at 8.00 in the morning litter picking. This goes on for two hours every day so you don't find a scrap of rubbish anywhere, after which they revert to strimming, clipping and other duties. In the evening, they are aided by an army of rabbits who pop out of their burrows and continue the good work well into the night, leaving their pellets as evidence.

There is a very green element to the park with plenty of recycling bins everywhere. Sustainability is particularly noticeable in the tented areas. Here the low-flow toilet and shower blocks have underground heating, using high efficiency condensing boilers and an automatic temperature control system so no heat is wasted. They have curved roofs, which blend into the landscape, and are covered with specially selected grasses, which will not cross-pollinate this unique protected area.

There are rain water harvesting tanks under the building that collect water from the roof and return it to hydrate this special living insulating layer. Solar panels provide water heating for the showers. It is good to be part of a system that respects the earth. And, just to emphasise that fact, around the park are billboards pointing out that the beach is not an ashtray and that plastic bottles will be around for hundreds of years before they eventually disappear from our oceans.

Day 4

The nets are getting to me! I am up at 5.00 a.m. this morning trying to get them finished. To my amazement I hear a van pull up outside and there is the security guard disposing of some rubbish that had been left outside one of the bins and redistributed by the seagulls. It is comforting to know security is patrolling regularly and checking on everything. They are easily recognizable with their blue shirts clearly labelled SECURITY and their clearly branded vans.

On our arrival, Trudy had given us a 24/7 number to ring in case of a medical emergency. This to me is very important because, with Mike being an insulin-dependent diabetic, there are occasions on which medical help is urgently needed. She explained that they will give you a doctor's number and will wait at the entrance to direct the doctor to the relevant caravan. It was very reassuring to have this information, with our family doctor being on the other side of the English Channel.

After a day finishing and fixing the nets, a trip into Perranporth, a snooze for Mike and delicious fish and chips from the on-site shop, washed down with a rose wine from the mini market, we decide to walk down to the beach through Penhale sands the most extensive dune system in Cornwall just five minutes from my front door.

I go into the bedroom to pick up a sweater and cannot believe my eyes. After a very, very hot day the Velcro suspending my precious nets is hanging in loops off the van walls. My brilliant plan has ended in ruins, but luckily not for long. My other daughter-in-law, Dani, comes up with the solution. Tomorrow the Velcro will be fixed using screws and cover plates. I am very lucky to have such a patient handyman - Mike.

Having solved another of life's little problems, we set off for the sea through the highest dunes I have ever seen. To say it is challenging is an understatement, but what fun! We get to the bottom just as the sun is setting and what a sight meets our eyes. The deserted beach literally stretches for miles and blends into an oblivion of surf spray mist. Even if the whole park was heaving at the peak of the holiday season, there would surely be peace and quiet down here. There is not a scrap of litter anywhere and Trudy had already told us that every working department at Perran Sands does three to four beach cleans a year. What an example to us all.

We walk along the deserted shoreline and climb back along the official concrete path, winding our way back to the caravan through parts of the park we didn't even know existed, ready to greet our first overnighters; the grandchildren.

Day 5

After a fun sleepover, I am up early for a game of football on a flat part of the dunes just behind the caravan and outside the park, where ball games are only allowed in designated areas. Allowances have to be made for Granny Jane whose running capabilities are limited and the direction in which the kicked ball goes can only be described as random. Mike sensibly stays in bed during this bout of frenetic activity. I make a mental note to engage a personal trainer on my return.

Having fallen down various rabbit holes, run miles and generally worked up a considerable appetite, I collect said husband and we all visit the Hub, where you can book for all available activities. These range from aqua jetting to fencing, crafting to roller skating, all reasonably priced and 50% off with the privilege card or in some cases free. The thirteen-year-old goes for archery and the eleven-year-old for recycled crafting.

Breakfast in Alfie, the VW camper van is great fun. Mike reminisces about the time he spent driving one in the sixties and the kids have fun pretending to drive. Off to archery for the first time in fifty years for Mike, it is a new experience for my grandson who takes to it like a duck to water. Confidently the youngster draws the bow and gives the target a great sprinkling of arrows. Formerly in the county team, Mike gives a good showing and between them they have some very creditable results.

The day is sweltering so a dip in the pool is called for. The outside pool is a great relief from the chlorine and we splash around for ages; the kids chasing each other underwater and pretending to be dragons and sharks, whilst Mike reads his Kindle.

The next activity involves Mike, for the first and last time. Whistling round the park on a bright red Go-Kart gets him involved - although he says he will never do it again due to the heavy uphill pedalling and the kids' driving skills, which create thrills and spills at every corner. Luckily, I had only booked a half hour slot as both Mike and I are now shattered.

Two minutes from the van is a huge sand dune where the kids and I decide to have lunch, leaving Mike to sleep off the excitement with his Kindle. By now the sand is so hot that the youngsters have to wear shoes and sun cream is lathered on every exposed millimetre of skin.

We toil to the top of the dune which gives us an unexpectedly comprehensive view of the park. I had hoped that the belly board would act as a sand sledge but that was not to be, the board sits solid as a rock at the top of the slope and refuses to move. We scoff our lunch and decide to go in search of greater mountains to climb.

I have since ordered coffin-tailed Rolla sledges for the older grandchildren and a plastic bum slider for the younger ones which should be great fun. I believe that quite a bit of speed can be built up on the Rolla sledge and the dunes are ideal. This will be a project for the next visit.

We now progress to the mega dunes that Mike and I had traversed the night before and scramble up and down humungous tracts of sand creating sand avalanches; giving every valley a name, the Grand Canyon, Death Valley, Deadman's Creek, and the Perrahari Desert. We are saved from death by our trusty water bottles and transported by imaginary camels across acres of unexplored territory full of hostile savages and wild beasts. Next time I must remember to bring a compass and we will make a map. We make it back to the caravan just in time to set off for the re-cycled crafting. Mike is snoring happily and will soon to be joined by the thirteen-year-old, who had been worn out by our amazing day.

A young blond ranger, who had recently completed a degree in biology and animal behaviour, is conducting the recycled activity. There are numerous ranger activities on offer during the week from nest box building to grass head creation and from bug hunting to crafting dream catchers. Happily, we convert the despised plastic water bottle into an octopus with the addition of woolly tentacles and googly eyes. This is followed by a beach collage which will be the first piece of artwork to be put up in the van. We are supposed to be doing it in a handy tepee nearby but it is simply too hot. As the sun goes down, people ebb and flow past us watching rubbish magically being transformed into art with liberal amounts of glue, paint and imagination. It is the end of a brilliant day…………

Day 6

Tomorrow we will be gone, but today is the turn of the two-year-old grandson to experience what Perran Sands has on offer.

The whole area is dotted with play parks, in fact just outside our caravan are two swings and a wooden motorbike. It is two-year-old's heaven. I can't wait to see him on the plastic bum slider in the dunes hurtling towards infinity with not a care in the world. He is at the stage of scrambling onto anything within reach with absolutely no fear or assessment of risk.

As it is, he comes to grief on a climbing frame and manages to hit the bridge of his nose with a mighty thwack. I rush into the restaurant to be given an enormous pile of ice, as he sits on the bar and howls. We are immediately offered medical assistance, but with my background we decline; it is, however, great to know it is so readily available. My grandson isn't that keen on having ice applied so in the end an ice lolly proves to be the answer which he is persuaded to apply to the affected part at regular intervals. No major harm done.

The kids' menu in the restaurant is awesome and again we sit in Alfie, the VW van, for lunch. The little chap spends a great deal of time driving us to imaginary places and seeing imaginary sights. All children are issued with crayons to colour in their menus and they then have the opportunity to have their works of art put up on the wall of fame. This activity absorbs a lot of fidgeting. I find it hilarious to watch adults come into the restaurant and want to explore the van but, not keen to be seen to be interested, observe from afar in a somewhat coy manner.

We have no time for swimming or Go-Karts that day, so taken up was the little chap with the caravan, the play areas and the dunes. Another day of wonderful memories has been created.

I could not let a day pass, however busy, without some 'net' activity. I grin to myself as I think how the meaning of 'net' has changed for me; how my priorities have altered after just seven days in a little tin box in Cornwall. When I arrived the importance of the (Inter) net was central to my existence; whether it was up or whether it was down. Now the crucial fact is whether the (curtain) net is up or down and I am more than happy with this fundamental change.

Mike fixes the Velcro and there is one last tweak I need to make, which is to neaten each end of each curtain. My plan is to seal the ends with a cigarette lighter. Having tried the procedure out on a piece of spare net with good results I graduate to the real thing. Running my lighter along the fabric edge, pouf, the nylon catches fire and before my very eyes the edge of the fabric resembles the seashore, wavy and brown. As so often in life, my instant solution is an instant disaster; back to the drawing board and the good old hem. I am looking at purchasing a very light sewing machine to keep "on board" as I can see there will be lots to do. Overall, with the Velcro secure and apart from the unhemmed edges, I am really pleased with the result of my labours. The butterflies make our van stand out from any other and I can now observe without being observed.

It is now time to pack up and go. As the park is renting out the van until my return in a couple of months, I stack all our possessions into the outdoor seating which is then padlocked. How glad I am that we have two seats. Because we live so far away I can leave quite a few woollies behind, including the fabulous knitted coat from the charity shop in Perranporth, for chilly evenings. I even take down the nets, as I want to finish securing the edges before letting them loose on the unsuspecting public.

The van was provided with a mop, sweeping brush, hand brush and pan. Next time I will bring my cordless vacuum cleaner with a hand-held unit incorporated into the handle making life a lot simpler. For now, I simply have to brush for England.

As I clean out our little nest I marvel how fast all this had happened, how lucky I am to have found the park, which fits our purpose, the perfect pitch, the van with which I am now deeply in love and Haven's excellent after-sales service, all of which we have experienced this week.

Day 7

As our car, loaded to the gunwales, pulls out of Perran Sands for the last time on this visit, it is without that hopeless feeling of bereavement that usually washes over me as I leave Cornwall. It has been replaced by the feeling that this is the start of a whole new chapter in my life. In two months' time, Mike and I will be back to cement our new relationship with the little tin box and play host to the family once more. Not only us, but we will be bringing our rescue dogs to complete the family menagerie.

I could not have done it without my amazing father who left me the inheritance, my incredibly understanding husband, a family who supported me every inch of the way and the Haven staff at Perran Sands, whom I could trust to guide me through the minefield that is buying a static caravan.

We, as a family, tend to make our own entertainments so the evening cabarets and shows were not for us. The amusement arcade was lovely and bright and airy but again, not on our 'to do' list.

There is a whole programme of events created for owners throughout the year; parties, outings, wine tastings, evenings in the Dune Bar and much more. I can't wait to join in and become a part of the Perran Sands' extended family.

Now that the book is almost finished it is time to christen our van. The name springs from the pages of one of my favourite books of all time, "The House at Pooh Corner," by A. A. Milne.

At the end of the book, when Christopher Robin is going to grow up and leave the forest, he and Pooh go to the 'Enchanted Place'. This is the place where they can play forever and to which they can return whenever they please, for magic is never very far away.

Our van is now 'The Enchanted Place' where you never quite know what will happen next.

Mike, proof reading this book suddenly looks up and says,
"You know why you didn't feel right with the van straight away?"
I shake my head,
"It was in the wrong place."
Mystery solved.

Work It Out In a Week: Buying a Static Caravan

Chapter 5
The Background to the Park

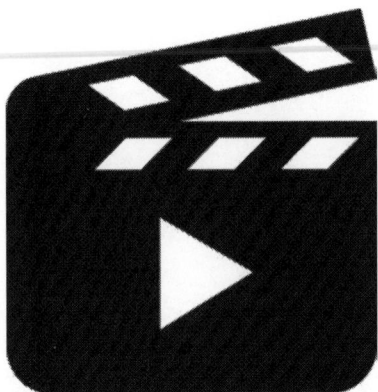

Perran Sands was established in 1947 and is celebrating its 70th anniversary in 2017.
In 2000, it was taken over by the Bourne Leisure group.

It is a self-catering holiday park with static caravans and chalets, with the touring area featuring caravans, tents, Super tents, Yurts, Safari tents and Geo-domes.

Perran Sands is unique being set within a Site of Special Scientific Interest (SSSI) and Penhale Dunes Special area of Conservation (SAC).

It is a beach front park and during June – September they have a beach hub cafe with surf and paddle board school. They welcome over 23,000 families who holiday with them each year and the park capacity reaches is excess of 5,500 guests at peak times.

Energy Saving and Sustainability issues

On the park, there has been an investment in five electric vehicles and one hybrid.

All venues and offices have now been fitted with LED lighting. The toilets in all amenity buildings have been fitted with motion-sensor lighting.

There are energy efficient boilers throughout the park and two of the touring amenity buildings have energy efficient boilers with solar. A combined heat and power unit (CPH) has been installed which converts gas to electricity to heat the pool and complex.

The Clubroom is now completely insulated and the Surf Bay Restaurant and swimming pool building have been reroofed to new efficiency standards.

Two eco amenity touring buildings have been created with curved grass roofs so that they blend in with the natural contours of the sand dune system. These are cedar clad with rain water harvesting to feed the green roof and were installed with low flow shower heads and low/dual toilet flush systems with under floor heating.

There are 50 recycling bays and in 2016 the recycling increased by 26% on 2015.

Perran Sands is a Member of the Energy Managers Association (EMA) They have saved 8% on electricity consumption in the first half of 2017 and monitor water daily to enable them to act on any leaks instantly. They continue to support Volunteer Cornwall with Beach Cleaning events, supplying free parking and removal of all the litter collected. Perran Sands sponsors Perranporth Surf Lifesaving Club with a contribution of £2,000 each year. In 2016, they raised £18,716 for Children in Need and donated £1,950 of carrier bag charges to the Marine Conservation Society. They hold a "Big Green Weekend" each year to educate their guests on sustainability and have also invested in 71 new energy efficient caravans for 2017.

Awards

David Bellamy Gold Plus Innovation Award 2015

Honeybee Friendly Award 2016

Cornwall Tourism Awards 2014/15 – Wildlife Friendly Business Award – Bronze 2015/2016 Silver

Investors in People Gold

Holiday Park of the Year Bronze 2014/2015

Holiday Park of the Year Silver 2016/2017

Commended wildlife friendly 2013/14 Bronze 2014/2015 Silver 2015/2016

GTBS Gold

The Perran Sands' inside story by general manager June Donnery

Our beach, ocean and sand dune wildlife is at the heart of the business, without it the product we offer would be diminished. This would impact directly on return visits and advocacy.

The team work tirelessly to litter pick. Attention to detail means the strandline habitat is left undamaged & prevents plastic from entering the ocean. Holidaymakers see the team leading by example and this helps to change behaviour.

We monitor Silver Studded Blue butterflies, Shore dock and Petalwort. We work with botanist Ian Bennallick to look at Shore dock populations. Butterfly transects are carried out. These are important as Penhale Dunes are the last site for Grizzled Skipper butterflies in Cornwall.

We support Exeter University PhD students who look into predation of Six Spot Burnet moths and how colour plays a role in their defence.

Records are passed to the environment records centre for Cornwall & isles of Scilly (ERCCIS) using Online recording for Kernow & Scillies (ORKs)

Perran Sands and the Cornwall Wildlife Trust signed a new Countryside Stewardship scheme in 2016 that runs for five years. This will fund habitat management work on the dunes. Work so far includes scrub removal, fencing to enable grazing and mowing of dune slacks.

Perran Sands have become partners in the £8m Heritage Lottery Fund / LIFE Dynamic Dunescapes – Raising Golden Sands Project. This shows a commitment to a five-year project running from 2018 to 2023. It is being run by The Wildlife Trusts, Natural England, The National Trust, Natural Resources Wales and Plantlife. The project aims to inspire and engage people, re-energise the dunes and create important new habitats. Perran Sands has committed its 110 ha of sand dune to the project.

We have created a new pond which is already home to diving water beetles and dragonflies and is the only permanent water body on the dunes. It is also used for pond dipping activities.

The yard to the rear of the park, with piles of composting vegetation, is home to grass snakes. Bird boxes cover the toilet blocks in the touring section and have residents in each one. Bug hotels are also located in this area and near reception, where there is a bird feeding station.

We lead activities for people of all ages around the park and special area of conservation (SAC). This helps to spark an interest in wildlife and the environment.

Activities include nest box building & pond dipping. Holidaymakers take their nest boxes home which encourage an interest in their local wildlife. They are also given advice on how to build ponds at home.

Perran Sands is a Cornwall Wildlife Trust Partner.

We fund Penhale Dunes Ranger and are part of the SAC Management group. Cornwall Wildlife Trust delivers countryside stewardship objectives set by Natural England on behalf of Perran Sands.

All the team support the Surfers Against Sewage Beach cleans.

Beach Front Boffins is a new set of four informative panels on coastal birds, flora and fauna, the shoreline and the ocean. The panels have been designed with children in mind and have a brass rubbing and quiz activity linked to them.

To tie Beach Front Boffins in with other activities we have the 'Dune Ranger Certificate'. If holidaymakers take part in four or more Nature Rockz activities they are awarded the Dune Ranger Certificate.

We have interpretation signs around the park to inform our guests on "doing the right thing" whilst they holiday with us; to value and respect our wonderful environment.

Our mascot dog Murphy has written a new and positive dog charter to encourage all that use our landscape to handle their animals responsibly.

In conclusion…………………..

What June has written has shown that what the guest sees at Perran Sands is only the tip of the iceberg. There is a depth of caring for the earth and its creatures that underpins all the park activities and sustains them into the future.

Never EVER give up!

You too can find your perfect pitch………………..

26549271R00050

Printed in Great Britain
by Amazon